200 Dirty Talk Examples: How to Dirty Talk Your Way to the Most Graphic, Mind-Blowing Sex of your Life

By Philip King

For KM, the dirtiest girl I know.

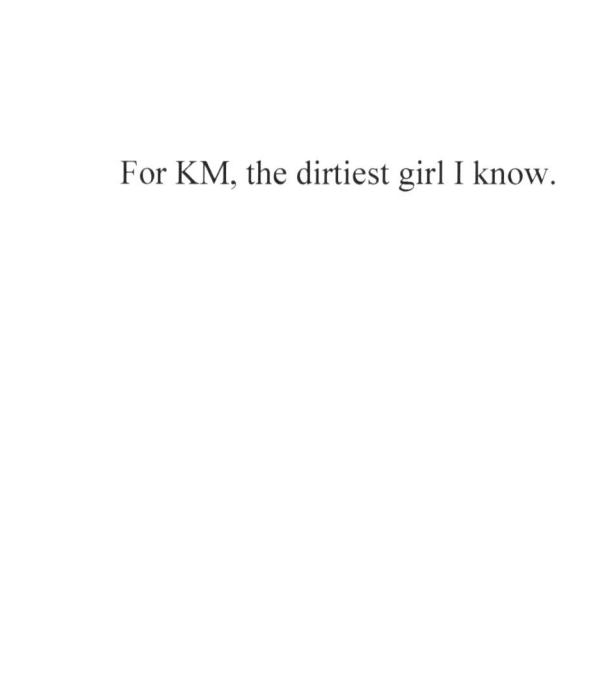

200 Dirty Talk Examples: How to Dirty Talk Your Way to the Most Graphic Mind-Blowing Sex of your Life

Introduction

So why should I learn to dirty talk?

- Enhance the sexual experience
- Communicate and give direction
- Foster openness and closeness

Getting started and breaking down barriers.

- Step one – bring it up innocently
- Step two – learn your vocabulary
- Step three – writing and typing it
- Step four – introduce outside of the bedroom
- Step five – transition to sex

It's in the delivery.

- Giggle attacks
- Eye contact
- Fake it 'til you make it
- Background music fills the gaps
- Warm up then ramp up
- Calibrate to your partner
- Just moan, damnit

The dirty talk phrases for every phase

- General guidelines
- Setting the stage
- Foreplay
- Intercourse

Orgasm
Post-coital

Conclusion

Introduction

The phrase "dirty talk" makes people uneasy. Visibly so. There is almost always a slight blush or facial tick of surprise and alarm when it comes up in conversation… which is rare in itself.

Some are embarrassed by it.

Some are intrigued by it but don't know how to get started with it.

Some embrace it, but can't talk about it freely with their friends.

Some are plain put-off by it out of a lack of awareness or shame.

Goodness, it's not debating the separation of church and state, people. It's just a part of our sexuality that is sadly underexplored and neglected. Those are all fine and natural reactions, but my aim in this book is to dispel them all and put people supremely at ease with dirty talk.

I find that people start warming to the idea once they discover that dirty talk doesn't have to consist of the exaggerated *"FUCK ME IN MY HOLE!"* of professional pornography.

In fact, dirty talk can be tender, gentle, loving, and serve an integral purpose in strengthening and growing a healthy relationship. It doesn't have to be dirty at all.

Intrigued?

Dirty talk can install confidence and openness in a relationship. It can foster communication. Taken altogether, dirty talk can enhance your sexual encounters and bring the most intense orgasms ever.

All you have to do is look to the popular media and even news. Sex is everywhere and it's unavoidable. I can see 7 nipples before I have my morning coffee.

We should feel free to shed the taboo and embarrassment of talking about dirty talk. If you're already having a sexual encounter with someone, you're about as vulnerable and open as you can be… so why not take that extra tiny step into opening your mouths and making sparks fly?

The overall legitimate utility of dirty talk (yes, I just used that phrase to describe whispering dirty nothings during sexual intercourse) combined with the powerful realization that a silent bedroom is the ultimate antiaphrodisiac leads us to only one logical solution: embrace the power of dirty talk.

Let's begin your journey to becoming the dirtiest mouth you know.

So why should I learn to dirty talk?

Let's get this out of the way immediately. There's absolutely nothing wrong or innately sinful with dirty talk. If used effectively, it can be a tool for delivering and receiving the most powerful orgasms and sexual encounters of your life. That doesn't sound so bad, does it? Unfortunately, popular media, for the amount of sex it depicts on a daily basis, tends to shame open sexuality and the expression of inner desires.

Perhaps because dirty talk contains the word "dirty." Perhaps because it embodies and represents non-vanilla sex, which tends to offend more conservative and religious sensibilities. Perhaps it's because culturally we like staying behind closed doors with our sexuality.

Or (more likely)…

Perhaps it's because our conception of dirty talk is informed by unrealistic and fake pornography. Perhaps it's because we simply have no idea how to do it or even broach the subject with our partner. Perhaps we're just too self-conscious and afraid of judgment.

Am I starting to strike a chord here?

Whichever the case, the buck stops *here* and the so should the stigma. Look around in popular media and the news. As I mentioned before, sex is everywhere. Turn on the television and watch any commercial. As a matter of fact, simply Google search "dirty talk," "dirty talk tips" or "how to dirty talk" and see how many results you get.

Within the stigma, there's clearly a market and a demand for more knowledge about the subject. It's almost a shame how secretive most people are about wanting to learn about things like this. But really… ladies, do you remember the first time you got your period, and how scary it was… and how run of the mill it seems now? Men, the same with your first erections?

Consider this book your first dirty talk period or boner! Once you dip your toe in, you'll look back and laugh at how tentative you were about it in the first place.

Now that we've *accepted the acceptance* of dirty talk, let's explore the benefits that you'll receive from it.

Enhance the sexual experience

First of all, it simply enhances the sexual experience for both parties by an order of magnitudes. This can't come as a surprise to anyone, and is the primary reason people seek to learn about dirty talk in the first place. Sex is great, but sex with bells and whistles is transcendent.

For each of our five senses – sight, touch, smell, taste, and of course sound – we have certain *pleasure triggers*. A typical trigger for the sense of smell might be something like smelling a delicious lasagna in the oven, and a typical trigger for the sense of sight might be seeing the lights on at home indicating that your beau is there.

A pleasure trigger is a stimulus that immediately arouses your sense of pleasure and excitement, and can enhance your mood and whatever you are currently engaging in. A pleasure trigger usually has a physical component and reaction too – a watering mouth and increased heart rate from the above examples.

Pleasure triggers translate obviously to sexual intercourse. Many things can serve to arouse us and give us pleasure directly or indirectly. You can become triggered into arousal and excitement by the sight of a lacy corset or silk sheets. You might be triggered by the touch of kneepads and the ground (you naughty girl, you). They evoke a mental reaction of arousal, and often an accompanying physical component – hardness, wetness, etc.

And here is where dirty talk enters the equation – as an auditory pleasure trigger. If we're engaging the rest of our five senses in pleasure during a sexual encounter, why wouldn't we use our mouths and audio? It just makes sense!

Incorporating dirty talk into dates, seduction, and sex can make for extreme anticipation and subsequent release. You can have the most powerful orgasms of your life, and the recipe to keep making it happen!

Communicate and give direction

Second, dirty talk is extremely functional, which is not a perspective many people realize. Dirty talk can be a subtle yet effective communication tool to tell your partner what you like, how you like it, and more importantly, what you don't like. It can direct your sexual encounters into mind-blowing pilgrimages.

Bonus if either sexual partner is into being commanded, or commanding…

Foster openness and closeness

Third, opening the flood gates of dirty talk will create a closer bond between you and your partner. Once you've given over to the dark and dirty side, you'll find that there's not much else that you would feel uncomfortable saying to your partner.

If you can communicate your deepest desires comfortably, then it's like a wall being smashed in terms of what you feel comfortable with in general.

Suddenly you don't feel so sheepish talking about the issue of washing the dishes when you told him last night to fuck your holes and treat you like a whore. This can easily translate to other aspects of your life, and lead to an overall personality change for the better.

You've said what you wanted to say, and the world didn't end, nor did you get judged into obligation. Self-consciousness can become a thing of the past, and that's a very empowering realization.

It's worth mentioning that auditory pleasure triggers generally differ between genders. If we take a moment to think about the different kinds of stimulation men and women want, this makes sense. When a man wants to become aroused, he will probably watch hardcore pornography with a focus on direct visuals and penetration. When a woman wants to become aroused, she will more often opt for erotica, erotic literature, or other forms of indirect stimuli.

What does this say about men and women?

For one, it says that we men are easy. We know what we want, and just want to be shown and told it. We want to hear dirty talk about what women want, how they want it, and how much they love it. Throw in a few moans otherwise, and a man's brain is filled for days. We want direct stimulation and don't want to be bothered by ancillary needs such as storyline or romance.

Women on the other hand are a bit more refined in what arouses them. They like to use their imaginations and create mental imagery. This is because their conception of amazing sex will include romance and love more often than not. This means that they want to hear more of a narrative and be whisked away by the sweet nothings that are whispered.

The difference between these approaches and preferences will become stark clear in the following chapters.

Getting started and breaking down barriers.

Even with the realizations that we've reached in the previous chapter, it can be tough to simply open your mouth and utter those things. Logic has nothing to do it with it, and self-consciousness and potential judgment everything.

We can have all the justification in the world to do something, but that's not what determines our actions in daily life… as many of us are far too familiar with.

Even if I give you the perfect phrases to whisper, they will be useless until you can actually work up to whispering or shouting them during orgasm.

Simply put, the first time you try anything new, you will feel that self-consciousness and adrenaline rush of uncertainty. It is unavoidable. But there are steps you can take to reduce those feelings and turn them into excitement and arousal.

Hell, you might even skip over a couple of the following steps because you've acclimated more quickly than you expected – and that's what I find with most people. The important thing here is that everyone moves along at their own pace of comfort, and no one can be expected to follow someone else's and move together exactly.

So if your partner is lagging, guess what… go back and help them!

Step one – bring it up innocently

First, talk about dirty talk with your partner. Bring it up innocuously and gauge their reaction to it. Tell them that a friend told you about it, and you were intrigued, so that the burden can be blamed on someone else. Or say that you read an article about it, saw a television piece on it, etc. You can also watch something together that has elements of dirty talk so the topic comes up independently of you.

Bringing it up this way gives you an out and plausible deniability so you can avoid self-consciousness and judgment. Your partner most likely will not be judging you, but this is an approach that helps you justify talking about it.

I would estimate that 99% of the time, your partner will be intrigued and agreeable to trying whatever you suggest in the name of spicing up bedroom relations. If they aren't, they might simply be in the same shoes you are – afraid of judgment and self-conscious about their sexuality. If that's the case, you need to move along slowly and emphasize that you are interested in exploring it.

You might need to bring the topic up more than once for it to truly implant in your partner's head.

If they are truly reluctant to give it a shot, there's not much you can do except continue to keep communication lines open and extoll the virtues of dirty talk.

Do *not* push them into something they don't want to try.

Step two – learn your vocabulary

Don't dive into using dirty talk during sex yet.

You need to focus on the two main components of dirty talk – *vocabulary, and action phrases*.

As you'll see, you will need to be comfortable and proficient with both of them. Get used to using various vocabulary words such as "cock," "pussy," "tight," "soaked," "fuck me" and so on. *Think* about how you can use them in your daily life to get over any prevailing stigma you might feel from them.

Roll them around your tongue and mouth them – you don't need to outright say or use them yet. You can do the same with action phrases such as "I'm going to," "spread yourself," "bend over," "pound me," and the like. Whisper them to yourself and become comfortable with them.

You are becoming a person who is a dirty talk expert, and that requires changing your mindset and expanding your comfort zones.

Make sure that you are also ridding yourself of your daily usage of lesser dirty talk words like "wiener," "dick," "vagina," and so on. Those are kiddy words. They have no place in dirty talk.

Step three – writing and typing it

Third, test these phrases and vocabulary out via text or instant messaging. Actually writing these out will be adrenaline-inducing for the first few times, but you'll find that the initial hurdle… is really the only hurdle there is. The first time is the hardest, and each time you use anything you'll be exponentially more comfortable with it. Once you see that there is no negative reaction, that's going to be a powerful piece of positive reinforcement to keep pushing the envelope!

If you need an intermediate step between steps two and three, I suggest seeking out an online chatroom geared towards cybersex and dirty talk. For some, this skirts a moral grey area, but it's in the name of love! Try out your phrases anonymously and without fear of retribution and judgment! The goal is just to get used to actually using them on someone, and seeing the proper context and reactions that people will have. You might even pick up a few tips while you're there.

Once you've mastered using your phrases and vocabulary via the written word, you can try trotting them out in person in the next step.

Step four – introduce outside of the bedroom

Fourth, now that you're comfortable with all the phrases and words and actually have used them to some degree, try using them in a joking manner with your partner *out loud… not during sex*. Take away the stigma and the embarrassment by saying everything with a wry smirk, and get used to saying the words and their reactions.

You'll get a chance for feedback, practice, and to discover what your partner particularly likes or does not like. Watch some amateur pornography for inspiration on how to use dirty talk naturally and organically. If you're still having trouble, try finding some audiobooks of erotica or erotic stories online – you can see exactly what kind of tone and inflection that you can use.

The goal in this step is to get used to saying the vocabulary and phrases with your partner orally to find out what they like and build comfort.

Step five – transition to sex

Finally, transition into the bedroom. At this point, you should have no issues saying that you want to say because you've already taken away the mystique of the words in other contexts. You should also realize at this point that there will be no judgment on your partner's part. This is key.

It will be slightly nerve-wracking because it is a new context, but you'll have these phrases at the tip of your tongue and instinctually realize when to use them for maximum arousal.

Start with moaning and groaning louder and more emphatically than normal.

Then continue by incorporating dirty talk phrases into your moaning and groaning. Practice makes perfect!

You may find that you have to do the majority of the leading and dirty talking when you first begin with your partner, so be prepared for it.

The wonderful part about dirty talk is that you have probably been playing a waiting game – that is, your partner didn't want to be the first person to bring it up, and is thankful that you did it. Discovering shared secret interests, especially those of the dirty nature, can be a huge aphrodisiac in itself.

It's in the delivery.

The phrase "It's not what you say, but how you say it" has rarely mattered more than with dirty talk. I can feed you the phrases to use (and I will later), but there are a few guidelines that we have to cover in the delivery of your dirty talk. Of course, part of this is practice and realizing what works for you and your partner.

Delivery is key for dirty talk because of the overall mood and tone you are seeking to cultivate.

Giggle attacks

First, we have to talk about giggling.

This is the first guideline for a reason. Everyone, me included, will occasionally suffer from giggle attacks from delivering dirty talk. There's not much I can say to prevent, but I can try to emphasize the mood-killing effect of it.

When you yourself giggle during the *delivery* of dirty talk, it potentially ruins the mood of the entire sexual experience.

Instead of having a transcendent set of orgasms, giggling imparts the mood of just fooling around and laughing… which is not how anyone would describe passion. The best orgasm you've ever had – I bet you weren't laughing before it. The steamiest, hottest sex you've had – I bet jokes weren't a component. We're aiming for raw, primal passion, and a case of the giggles simply breaks that path.

The next time you're on the verge of giggling during your delivery, just bite your tongue until the moment passes.

And giggling from *receiving* dirty talk from your partner? Now that's a crushing blow in two ways: to their confidence in their dirty talk skills, and to the mood that they are trying to cultivate. Avoid that at all costs. In the same vein, never criticize their dirty talk or make them feel bad about it until after the session.

Eye contact

Eye contact is a powerful tool in all walks of life, so it's only natural that it should be paired with expert dirty talk. Whenever possible, pair dirty talk with eye contact, regardless of whether you are receiving or delivering it.

If you are in a situation (or position) in which you aren't facing each other at the moment but feel the need to deliver some dirty talk, take a moment's pause from whatever you doing, seek eye contact (or outright grab their face), and say it. It's a power move that will enhance the words coming out of your mouth, and make your partner want you that much more… and return to the task at hand with renewed vigor and lust.

Whispering dirty talk into someone's ear from behind or from the front is one of the only acceptable times where eye contact would not necessarily enhance the phrases.

If you find that you have trouble with eye contact in general walks of life, I have a practice tip for you. Put on a pair of sunglasses, and take a stroll around your block. Make eye contact with people that you walk across with impunity, because they can't see your eyes. It's like viewing them through a one-way mirror! Notice how many people make only a spit-second of eye contact, or avoid it altogether.

This exercise is to realize that eye contact is easier than you think, and that other people also have trouble with it.

Fake it 'til you make it

As with many things in life, people will become comfortable with dirty talk only when they can sense that you are also comfortable with it. For example, if someone is extremely self-deprecating and depressed, that makes the people around him uncomfortable because they simply don't know how to react.

Dirty talk embodies that feeling of mutual comfort. If your partner can sense that you are uncomfortable with the things you are saying, it will diminish the experience and decrease their comfort and enjoyment levels intensely.

It's unavoidable for us to 100% comfortable and confident in our dirty talk skills the first few times around, so my advice here is simply to fake that comfort and confidence until it becomes real. Whisper or demand things in a strong and clear tone of voice, and don't let on that you are way out of your comfort zone… because then you will take them out of theirs.

Don't utter something then ask if that was okay or embarrassing.

Own it.

Whisper, state, demand, and scream confidently!

Background music fills the gaps

Even though this is obviously a book on the virtues of dirty talk, I should make it clear that I'm not suggesting that your sexual encounters be like a Gilmore Girls episode – non-stop chatter and banter.

Playing music in the background will help reduce the need to fill the space with dirty chatter. It's also a good intermediate step for beginners, as having the background noise will make novices less self-conscious about what they're saying.

At first, turn the music on loudly so your partner will barely hear your words, but you get acclimated to using them during actual sex. Gradually turn the music volume down, and you've just gradually conditioned yourself to be less self-conscious with dirty talk.

On another note, playing background music during sex is great for setting the mood and tone of the sex itself... which will influence the type of dirty talk that you whip out.

Boyz 2 men? Get ready for a steamy session with lots of slow kissing and grinding.

Rammstein? Well...

Warm up then ramp up

Just like most sexual experiences, dirty talk should start more slow and tame... and then ramp up to dirty and downright filthy when the intensity of the sex picks up.

During any sexual encounter, there are necessary phases of arousal that we all go through. This is both a mental and physical process that culminates in an erection or adequate lubrication. Sometimes we go through it quickly and even skip a phase or two, but more often than not, we proceed through each stage methodically.

It's a time-tested process that heightens arousal and sets an individual's mood. If you are disturbed from that process that you are used to, you risk being taken out of the mood entirely.

You wouldn't try shoving your cock into her while she's barely wet, would you? You can't shove your mindcock into her brainpussy when it's barely lubed up either.

Skew to using more tender and gentle dirty talk at first, and save your filthy mouth for later when your partner will be able to appreciate it the most. This segues into my next point nicely.

Calibrate to your partner

As I discussed before, everyone has their set pattern and phases of arousal that they go through during a sexual encounter. Some people go through them quickly and are ready for sex at the drop of a hat, while others are slow starts and might need 15 minutes of foreplay to truly get into the mood.

The same variance applies to the types of dirty talk that people like. Some like it sweet, and some like it rough. Some might feel degraded, and some might want more degrading. Some want to be your slave, and some want to dominate you with a choke collar. There's nothing wrong with any of those – the only wrong thing is if you don't figure out which style works best for you and your partner.

It's up to you to discover you and your partner's optimal blend of dirty talk, and the easiest way to do so is to use a wide variety of dirty talk phrases and pay attention to your partner's verbal and non-verbal response. That will help you determine what really makes sparks fly, and what your go-tos should be.

Be careful with degrading dirty talk, as it has been shown to sometimes make women feel more emotionally distant from their partners, which is of course the opposite effect you want to have.

A final important part of calibrating to your partner is having a post-mortem discussion about what went well, what you each liked, and what should never be used again. Unsurprisingly, communication is key!

Just moan, damnit

If you're having sex right, sometimes you won't have a clear enough head to even form words in your mind.

So in lieu of dirty talk, oftentimes you should make an effort to moan and react effectively to your partner's actions. Any type of vocalization is going to enhance the experience, and sometimes a primal series of moans and whimpers can get the point across more succinctly and clearly than a well-placed "I want you inside of me."

Focusing on reacting will make you more present and in the moment with the experience, while some dirty talk practitioners can become slightly distant because they are focused on thinking about the next phrase to whisper.

Again, this is a good intermediate step for beginners to small talk. Simply breaking the sound barrier can be transformative, and moans and groans are easier to let slip and test the waters than dirty talk.

Finally, as I mentioned before, you don't actually have to respond to the questions that your partner might ask you during dirty talk.

"You like that?" *"Why, yes, I enjoy it very much, thanks."*

A lot of them are rhetorical in nature, and don't need a response for the intended effect. But you could always moan in acknowledgement, which would be a good way to get your feet wet, as well as show your appreciation of their dirty talk.

The dirty talk phrases for every phase

Finally, what you've been waiting for. When most people want to learn about dirty talk, I find that they usually just want exact creative and sexy phrases that they can borrow. I have no problem with this, as I've learned many phrases from others as well.

We all need a baseline to start with before we can really discover our true dirty talk personality and character.

General guidelines

1. Describe how they are making you feel by what they are doing to you in that moment. Make it personal, that they are the ones affecting you and only them.
2. Direct them – command, ask, beg, demand, or plead. Also, add "please" to many dirty talk phrases.
3. Narrate your actions. Tell them what you are doing, or what you are going to do to them.
4. Praise them. Be specific, and focus on their physical attributes. Many people's self-esteem is wrapped up in their physical appearance, so if you praise them, you are simultaneously building their confidence as

well as dirty talking. When someone is more confident about their body and has high self-esteem, they'll be more likely to explore new thing and be open – this can only work in your favor.
5. Talk in terms of possessions. You are hers, she is yours. Your cock is hers, her pussy is yours. Etc.
6. You don't have to actually answer a question they pose in their dirty talk. Many are rhetorical. As long as you acknowledge it or even moan to it, that is sufficient.

As you'll see, these six guidelines will be present in almost of all the dirty talk phrases I give you in this book.

For ease of digestion and visualization, I've grouped my dirty talk phrases into a few distinct phases. They run the gamut of when you could use them related to a sexual encounter, from days to weeks of teasing, to the actual encounter, during the orgasm, and afterwards. I'll educate you on the goals and tones you should be using for each phase.

Most of these phrases are fairly unisex and can be used without regard to gender or sexual orientation… and they are easily altered to fit your needs otherwise.

Setting the stage

This is the phase before you even see your paramour. This might be through texting, emailing, chatting, or even over the phone. The point here is to drive anticipation and hint at the promise of what's to come later. You can do this throughout the day, or week even, to make them hunger for you. The trick in setting the stage is to talk in future terms of what you want them to do to you, and what you want to do to them.

Have the mindset of trying to lure your partner over immediately – what would you say to tempt them? Imagine getting a text or email like this at work and the hungry reaction that you'll create.

1. I want you so bad
2. God I miss feeling you
3. You are going to feel so good inside me
4. I miss feeling your cock/pussy
5. I want you to lick my cock/pussy right now
6. I am going to pound you raw
7. I am going to drink all of your cum
8. I can't get enough of you
9. I need to taste you right now
10. I'm hard/wet just thinking about you
11. You make me so hard/wet

12. You drive me crazy
13. I dreamt about fucking you last night
14. I can't wait for you to spread me
15. I can't wait to spread you
16. I can't wait to fuck you from behind
17. I can't stop thinking about how you moan
18. I can't stop thinking about your pussy/cock
19. I am going to fill you up with my cum
20. How do you want to fuck me on Saturday?
21. How much cum are you going to give me on Saturday?
22. I don't want to wait for your cock/pussy
23. Only you can fuck me right
24. My pussy/cock aches for you
25. Tell me how you're going to fuck me
26. Fuck me please?
27. You're the tightest/biggest

28. I want to taste you now.

29. I love how you look at me when we fuck

30. Your pussy/cock is mine

Foreplay

For the purposes of this book, I'm counting foreplay as the moment your lips meet, and including everything until actual penetration. This includes oral and manual stimulation. Foreplay is all about teasing and increasing the anticipation for the main event. Focus on your partner and how they are making you feel, while hinting that the main event is going to blow your mind because of the anticipation you've had.

Have the mindset that you are in the desert and they are your oasis – you just can't get enough of them, and they can do no wrong. Make them feel amazing about themselves, and they will want to reciprocate physically.

1. You feel so good

2. Your smell is intoxicating

3. You feel amazing

4. You're so sexy/hot

5. I could do this all day

6. I love when you [fill in the blank]
7. Your skin feels so good
8. Your lips are so soft
9. Bite me
10. Spank my ass
11. Use your nails on me
12. Feel how hard/wet you make me
13. Just looking at you makes me hard/wet
14. You drive me crazy
15. Fuck my face
16. Strip now
17. Pull my hair
18. Dominate me
19. What do you want me to do?
20. Lie back, it's my turn
21. You look so hot sucking my cock
22. I want you in my mouth

23. You're so tight
24. You taste so good/sweet
25. You're so hard
26. Your pussy/cock tastes so good
27. Shove your tongue in me
28. Grab my cock and play with my balls
29. Tell me what to do
30. Gag on it
31. Make me gag
32. Rub your clit now
33. Can I put your cock in my mouth please?
34. Do you like that?
35. You have a nice load in there for me? [while grabbing his cock]
36. Everything about you turns me on
37. Kiss/suck my cock/pussy/clit
38. Your pussy/cock is mine

39. My cock/pussy is yours.
40. Am I being a good/bad girl?
41. Make me beg
42. Tease me
43. Don't tease me, just do it
44. You can have anything you want
45. Feel how ready I am [take his/her hand and lead it to your genitals]
46. You want to fuck me, don't you
47. Wrap your legs around me
48. You want to feel my cock in you?
49. I can't wait to be inside you
50. I need you inside me
51. Please?

Intercourse

Of course, intercourse counts as any form of penetration. Since this is the main event, talk about how you've waited eagerly for this, and that it's living up to all of your expectations. Talk about the actual thrusting and the mechanics that you enjoy behind it. Talk about how passionately you want the sex to be.

Try having the mindset that every thrust is mind-blowing, and that you can barely stop from orgasming from their touch. It's not true of course, but projecting such passion will turn your partner into an echo chamber.

1. Don't stop pounding me
2. Make me scream
3. Your pussy is so warm/tight
4. Your cock is so hot/big
5. You're filling me up
6. Fuck me harder
7. You feel so tight
8. Right there
9. Deeper
10. Only you can fuck me like this
11. Only you know how I love it
12. Give me that cock/pussy
13. I'm going to fuck you until you break
14. May I come?
15. You make me feel so full

16. Fuck that feels so good
17. That cock feels so good in my pussy
18. That's my good/bad girl
19. Say my name
20. Flip over and spread your pussy
21. Look at me
22. You look amazing spread under me/bent over
23. Choke me
24. I love feeling you inside me
25. Do you like that?
26. You are so hot
27. You drive me wild
28. I want to make you cum
29. Make me cum
30. I'm going to watch you cum
31. You're so deep
32. Do you like it deep?
33. I need you
34. I've been thinking about this all day
35. You're going to make me cum so hard
36. You like when I spread for you?
37. I'm going to suck you until you come

38. Ride me harder
39. You're my naughty girl
40. Bend over, slut
41. I love fucking you
42. Lick it clean
43. I'm going to clean you clean
44. You're so hard inside me
45. Moan for me
46. You're driving me crazy
47. I'm going to fuck you until you can't walk
48. I'm so fucking wet
49. Beg me
50. You own me
51. Take it all
52. You're my fucktoy now
53. Make me your fucktoy
54. You can do anything you want to me
55. Fuck my cunt
56. Spread your pussy lips
57. Tell me what you want
58. You're making me shake
59. Fuck me raw

60. Fuck me from behind
61. Make it hurt
62. Do you have any idea what you're doing to me?
63. I love your [fill in the blank]

Orgasm

This is where it's all been leading to. This is where you find your sense of relief, and the culmination of everything you've anticipated of your partner. Express it! Talk about how long you've wanted this, and that your partner is so irresistible that you simply couldn't help yourself. Cumplay is a big fetish for both genders, so having it inside, outside, on the woman's chest, in the mans' hair – someone is going to thoroughly it any way you do it.

Your mindset here should be that your orgasm is from your partner, by your partner, and solely for your partner.

1. I'm going to fill you up
2. Fill me up
3. I'm coming
4. Don't stop until you're empty
5. Come all over my cock
6. Take every drop
7. I'm coming all over your cock

8. I can't hold back any longer
9. I can't resist your cock/pussy
10. I can't take it anymore
11. Don't stop until I cum
12. You're going to make me cum
13. Give me your cum
14. Never stop, don't stop
15. I want to watch you come
16. Let's come together
17. Watch me cum for you
18. Can I come sir?
19. Watch me come for you
20. Come for me
21. Make me drip
22. Come in my mouth
23. I can't stop coming for you
24. Take it all
25. Look what you're doing to me
26. Shoot it deep inside me
27. I want to swallow you
28. Make my pussy scream
29. Where do you want me to come?

30. Come inside me

Post-coital

This is the phase after you catch your breath from the amazing orgasm that you just had due to your newfound dirty talk skills. They've heightened your experience and left you a sweaty mess. All you can do now is lament that it was over too soon, and look to setting the tone for the next session. Take this opportunity to praise your partner, talk about what you loved about the experience you just shared, and what you are looking forward to for the next one.

Your mindset here should be that you're sad that it was over so soon, but despite that, you can barely move from the orgasm.

1. You're so amazing/That was amazing
2. You're mine
3. I'm yours
4. Look what you did to me
5. I can't help myself around you
6. We're going to go again in 5 minutes
7. Make me beg for more
8. I can't control myself around you
9. How did you do that?
10. Next time, you can do whatever you want to me

11. You look so good full of my cum
12. I love you freshly fucked
13. I'm your toy, do whatever you want to me
14. I've been thinking about that for days
15. How long until you're ready for round 2?
16. Don't make me wait to fuck me again
17. You made me shake
18. You made me numb
19. Oh my God… (keep repeating this)
20. I need more of you
21. I love fucking/pounding you
22. Let me lick you clean
23. I can't feel my toes
24. You made me come so hard I'm shaking
25. Only you can fuck me so good
26. Your pussy/cock is amazing
27. Did you like being fucking used (like a fucktoy)?
28. You broke me
29. I'm going to be sore tomorrow
30. You're the best I've ever had

Conclusion

We've done it. We've made it through.

At this point, hopefully I've opened your eyes to the fact that dirty talk really doesn't have to be dirty. It can be whatever you want to make of it, and whatever fits your sense and sensibilities. It just makes sense to fully engage all five of your senses and fly to the greatest orgasms you've ever had.

It took a series of powerful realizations – that sex is right in front of our faces, that dirty talk is not inherently evil, and that dirty talk has multiple amazing purposes – to really open ourselves up to the benefits of dirty talk. We've defeated inner demons that prevent us from saying what we feel and have opened Pandora's Box.

I truly hope that you've found value in this book. Remember that dirty talk is a mindset, one that you can easily gain if you take the leap of faith with me and follow the steps I lay out. Doubt no more and discover what you've been missing from your life!

Sincerely,
Philip King

P.S. If you enjoyed this book or can at least see yourself using some of the phrases within, would you be so kind as to leave me a review on Amazon? I would appreciate it so much! Thank you!

Made in the USA
Lexington, KY
29 April 2015